THE ULTIMATE FOOD CLEANSE BOOK

A 30-Day Meal Plan to Detox Your Body, Lose Weight and Transform Your Body for Enhanced Energy

GODWINS INKLINE

THE ULTIMATE FOOD CLEANSE BOOK

...to Michael Eson

Copyright

No part of this book is allowed to be reproduced in any form without approval from the author.

Table of Content

CHAPTER 1

Introduction

An increasing number of people suffer from chronic health issues related to poor diet and lifestyle habits in the modern world. These include obesity, type 2 diabetes, high cholesterol, heart disease, and autoimmune disorders, among others. Pharmaceutical drugs provide temporary band-aid solutions without addressing root causes – our nutritionally-lacking processed food diets and high-stress sedentary lifestyles. Is there a way to eat and live that enables our bodies to function optimally and self-heal? That is the premise of the Clean Food Reset – a 30-day elimination diet that removes inflammatory modern foods to allow your body to rebalance and thrive in the way nature intrinsically designed.

The Clean Food Reset draws inspiration from the Paleo diet, which mimics the food groups and ingredients available in the era of cavemen. Our hunter-gatherer ancestors foraged vegetables, fruits, nuts, seeds, eggs, fish and meat. They moved constantly and did not suffer from today's chronic illnesses. Though we cannot fully replicate their lifestyle, we can use the evolutionary template as a baseline for identifying problematic modern foods. The Reset removes grains, dairy, legumes, added sugars, processed vegetable oils, chemical additives and artificial ingredients for one month. What remains is a clean, whole food diet centered around vegetables, fruits, nuts/seeds, protein and healthy fats.

These simple ingredients may seem limiting at first. But the Detox guarantees satiation and satisfaction, once initial withdrawal pangs fade. You will likely experience improvements in digestion issues, skin conditions, mental health, sleep quality and energy levels. Stubborn excess weight also starts dropping off. The benefits arise from both removing inflammatory foods that disrupt body processes and flooding your system with a potent barrage of micronutrients lacking in modern diets. Your tastebuds become resensitized to natural flavors. You stop constantly craving salty, oily, sugary junk foods. Feeling lighter and healthier becomes addictive!

What Clean Food Reset Diet is and its Benefits

The Clean Food Reset is a 30-day elimination diet that removes inflammatory modern foods, allowing your body to rebalance and function optimally. It takes inspiration from the Paleo diet, which replicates the food groups available to our ancient hunter-gatherer ancestors. Humans evolved eating vegetables, fruits, nuts, seeds, eggs, fish and meat while constantly active outdoors. Chronic disease was nonexistent back then. Though we cannot fully replicate caveman life in the modern world, we can use it as a Paleo-inspired template for identifying problematic inflammatory foods in our diets today.

The Clean Food Reset cuts out grains, dairy, legumes, processed foods, sugar and vegetable oils. These ingredients disproportionately disrupt digestion, gut health and metabolic processes, promoting systemic inflammation. Inflammation is the common root cause behind modern epidemics like obesity, heart disease, diabetes and autoimmunity. We ingest it daily for years through processed carbs, industrial seed oils and chemical additives until illness takes hold. The Reset presses control-alt-delete on the inflammation spiral. It floods your system with micronutrients from vegetables, fruits and healthy fats instead, giving cells what they need to function and heal optimally.

Benefits show up shockingly fast, as soon as bloating and water weight flush out in the first week. Bowel movements regulate, skin clears up and brain fog lifts without all the gut-disrupting ingredients. Stubborn body fat starts dropping off quickly too. But the real magic happens deeper down over 30 days as inflammation subsides systemwide. Gut health strengthens, stabilizing everything from hormone balance to mood. Autoimmune conditions, asthma, acne, diabetes and fertility issues all benefit from the anti-inflammatory effects. With cleaner eating, you effortlessly normalize weight as your body sheds lbs trying to protect itself from the daily damage of modern foods. Equally vital, tastebuds heal from constant overload so veggies and natural flavors excite them again. Cravings shift from salty, oily indulgences towards the saver goodness in produce and clean protein. You break out of the exhausting reward-punishment diet cycle because healthy food makes you feel too good!

The physical benefits compel you towards maintaining these habits long after the 30 Day Reset ends. Mental and emotional health improve too with balanced blood sugar and a reset dopamine system. In our stressed-out, hyperconnected society, that heightened sense of calm, focus and joy transduces into being more present for relationships and success at work or school. When healthy vitality becomes your steady baseline, life's challenges feel far more manageable. Lastly, the identity shift cannot be ignored – you stop being the sick, overweight person and step firmly into a body and mind healing itself with the magic of real food. Quite simply, you learn how good your life can feel minus years of self-inflicted inflammation holding you back!

The Approved and Non-Approved Food Groups

The Clean Food Reset is not a punishing, restrictive fad diet – it simply strips away modern inflammatory foods allowing your body to heal and thrive. The approved list focuses on ancestral whole foods filled with nutrients, enzymes and beneficial compounds. Plants make up the foundation, with fresh low-sugar fruits and a rainbow of non-starchy vegetables packed with antioxidants and phytonutrients. High quality proteins from pasture-raised animals raised on their natural diets provide satisfying nutrition. Raw nuts and seeds or their minimally processed butters add anti-inflammatory fats along with fiber and crunch. Rounding it out are beneficial seasonings like apple cider vinegar, garlic, onions and minerals salts. These whole ingredients form the baseline of what humans evolved eating for millennia while constantly active outdoors before chronic disease took hold.

1. Non-starchy vegetables - This is the foundation of the Clean Food Reset diet. Load up on leafy greens, broccoli, cauliflower, asparagus, peppers, mushrooms and more. They provide a potent dose of antioxidants, fiber, vitamins and minerals to heal inflammation, digestion issues and nutrient deficiencies.

2. Fresh fruits - Stick to mostly low sugar berry options and green apples or pears, which balance

their fructose with nutrients. Portion tropical fruits carefully for their higher sugar content. Fruit provides enzyme and phytonutrient support for the Reset.

3. Clean proteins - Grass-fed meat, wild caught seafood, pasture-raised poultry and eggs offer excellent protein on the Clean Food Reset diet. They satiate efficiently while providing iron and essential fatty acids like Omega 3s reduce inflammation.

4. Healthy fats - Focus on anti-inflammatory fats from avocado, olive oil, nuts, seeds and their butters. Coconut oil is great for high heat too. Fats slow digestion, buffer blood sugar spikes and help absorb fat soluble vitamins and antioxidants.

5. Herbs, spices & vinegar - Boost flavor generously with garlic, onions, vinegar, lemon, herbs and spices, which provide antioxidants along with taste.

Apple cider vinegar has additional gut and digestion benefits.

Non-Approved Food Groups

The non-approved list targets modern foods introduced by industrial food processing which disproportionately drive inflammation, poor digestion and nutritional deficiencies. The usual suspects top this list – grain products like cereals, breads and pasta made from genetically modified wheat, corn and soy, many of which spike blood sugar higher than actual sugar. While whole ancient grains can be carefully reintroduced after the Reset, modern hybridized grains tend to trigger inflammation, autoimmunity, brain fog and stubborn weight gain. Next come all dairy products, even full fat Greek yogurt and cheese, which contain difficult to digest sugars and proteins. Legumes like beans, lentils and peanuts provide beneficial nutrients but often provoke digestive distress with lectins and phytates. Less obvious offenders are vegetable and seed oils now ubiquitous in packaged goods and restaurant cooking, their fragile polyunsaturated fats oxidizing easily into inflammatory free radicals. Finally there are chemical additives like preservatives, artificial sweeteners, colors and flavors that alter gut bacteria negatively. During the 30 days, even approved sweeteners like maple syrup and honey should be minimized to reset tastebuds and blood sugar regulation.

1. Grains - Wheat, corn, rice, cereal, pasta, etc. They spike blood sugar, are often inflammatory and contain anti-nutrients like gluten, lectins, phytates limiting nutrient absorption. Allow inflammation to heal first before carefully reintroducing properly prepared ancient grains.

2. Dairy - Inflammatory for most people due to sugars, hormones and dairy proteins. Reintroduce goat or sheep products later only if no reaction.

3. Beans & legumes - Lectin and phytic acid content makes them hard to digest, promoting inflammation, gas and bloating. Later retest soaked, sprouted or fermented legumes.

4. Processed foods - Reset tastebuds and cravings by avoiding artificial sweeteners, flavors, colors, preservatives and inflammatory seed oils found in almost all convenience & junk foods.

5. Sugary foods - Resets elevated insulin and leptin hormones. Satiates efficiently without triggering sugar rollercoaster. Allows any candida overgrowths to heal so probiotics can repopulate.

6. Alcohol & coffee - Eliminate as both sensitivities and dependencies surface. Later reintegrate alcohol in moderation and only low-acid coffee variants if no inflammatory reaction.

That sums up the approved nutrient-dense whole food groups and excluded inflammatory modern foods on the Clean Food Reset diet. Base meals on produce, clean proteins and fats while omitting grains, dairy, processed items and sugar during the 30 days. Stay hydrated with plenty of water and herbal teas as well. Then slowly reintegrate approved ancient grains, fermented dairy, legumes, coffee and alcohol later only if no inflammatory reactions surface.

By removing this broad group of common yet evolutionarily mismatching modern foods for just 30 days, profound improvements in energy, body composition, chronic conditions and quality of life emerge for the over 80% of people suffering from inflammation-driven issues. As the dominant whole food groups – plants, animals raised on their natural diets and minerals – replace processed items, the body can finally absorb the nutrients, enzymes and phytochemicals essential for every biochemical process. Cells begin functioning optimally, relaying messages properly between digestion, hormones, neurotransmitters, metabolism and organs. Systemic inflammation driving chronic issues naturally resolve when not assaulted daily. With better cellular communication, your body effortlessly sheds excess weight trying to protect itself from the daily damage of modern foods. Equally vital, tastebuds heal from constant overload so vegetables, fruits and clean protein sources become delicious again. This push towards self-care transforms not just physical health but mental and emotional balance too.

Preparing for the Program

Setting Yourself Up for Success

Preparation is the key to effectively make it through the 30-day Clean Food Reset without falling prey to cravings, hunger and temptation. Follow this prep guide to set yourself up for success before embarking on the elimination diet.

1. Pantry Purge - Clear out all non-compliant foods from your kitchen like pasta, cereal, chips, cookies, dairy milk, soda, juices, alcohol and convenience meals. Having these trigger foods accessible will sabotage the program. Consider donating unopened items.

2. Meal Plan - Create a meal plan for the full 30 days incorporating approved breakfasts, lunches, dinners and snacks. Include lots of variety mixing proteins, veggies and healthy fats to prevent boredom. Prep recipes, grocery

lists and grab-n-go options like hard boiled eggs as well.

3. Stock Up - Shop farmers markets and grocery stores for produce, proteins and pantry staples like nuts, seeds, nut butters, eggs, avocados, olive oil and vinegar. Having Reset-friendly ingredients on hand prevents falling off plan when hunger strikes.

4. Wash Produce - Give fresh fruits and veggies a vinegar bath to remove pesticides and wax so your compromised detox organs don't get overburdened.

5. Food Prep - Chop veggies and pre-portion meat for easy cooking every few days. Stock snack drawers with cut up crudité, berries and nuts. Have compliant grab-n-go options handy for on-the-go.

6. Switch Out - Swap pantry basics to Reset-friendly alternatives like ghee for butter,

coconut aminos for soy sauce and unsweetened coconut or almond milk for dairy milk.

7. Restock Staples - Make sure to have coconut oil, olive oil, balsamic vinegar, garlic, lemons, herbs and spices on hand. They provide flavor diversity helping you stick to clean eating.

8. Hydrate - Stock up on sparkling water, herbal tea and water enhancers like lemon and lime slices or fruit infusers. Proper hydration is key as detox symptoms can intensify if you get dehydrated.

9. Start Moving - Prepare your body for enhanced nutrition absorption by starting to exercise before the program begins. This limits detox intensity and boosts results.

10.   Social Support - Share your Reset plans with friends, family and co-workers. Their

support improves accountability and makes saying "no" to peer pressure easier.

Embarking on an elimination diet feels daunting, but proper physical and mental preparation smoothens the transition's intensity. The upfront effort makes sticking to approved foods for 30 days much easier. Follow this prep checklist to clear out inflammatory items, stock up on Reset-friendly foods and create an encouraging support circle. Combined with the motivational and scientific guidance within the Clean Food Reset book, you are set up for success in reclaiming health, energy and body composition.

Chapter 2

Week 1 on the Clean Food Reset

Embarking on any elimination diet brings an adjustment phase before the numerous health benefits set it. The first week of the Clean Food Reset sees the biggest physical and mental shift as years of sugar dependence, unhealthy cravings and inflammation buildup start getting cleared out. Know that the intensity will pass, aided by the right coping strategies. Arm yourself with the foreknowledge that Days 3 through 5 often feel the most challenging.

As the first 72 hours pass without inflammatory foods, blood sugar surges, addiction cues and negative emotions can surface. Headaches, nausea, body aches, early waking or insomnia and fatigue often arrive as years of physiological gunk starts releasing. These symptoms subside as toxins clear out so view them as temporary healing crises. Limit vigorous training this first week to prevent feeling depleted. Gentler movement like walking, yoga or pilates supports natural detox pathways opening up instead.

Cravings and mood swings may catch you off guard with their intensity due to hormonal changes. The usual comfort foods triple down on hijacking your happy brain chemicals during this time so just know it will pass sooner than you expect. Initially it takes concerted willpower so deploy every clean eating trick you know – carrot sticks, big salads, lemon water, brushing your teeth after meals. Distraction is invaluable – walk outdoors, call a friend, immerse in a hobby, organize your pantry again. The slightest hunger pang can also trigger overeating approved foods, so watch portions and eat every 4 to 5 hours to stabilize blood sugar. Incredibly, just a few days in, irritation and desires fade as your body adapts hormonally to consistent nutrition all day.

Stock up on satiating proteins, healthy fats and insoluble fiber which does wonders to eliminate cravings. When one hits, ask yourself, "Am I just mouth hungry or actually stomach hungry?" More often insatiable mouth hunger drives cravings, not genuine appetite. Drink some water first, then focus on a task for 15 minutes before reassessing if you need sustenance. Often the intensity dies down.

Social events trip up folks starting elimination diets, so prepare excuses in advance to politely decline tempting food. Say you're on a health cleanse ordered by your doctor, clarify it's a temporary reset not a permanent diet, shift focus to the restaurant's menu options you can enjoy, or offer to bring your own compliant dish. Most people respect when you confidently state it is an important reboot for your body.

Digestive issues are very common the first week with bowel movement inconsistencies, initial bloating and gas. This is just the bad stuff clearing out without daily influx of gut irritants. Support the process by staying hydrated with herbal tea and water. Add gentler herbs like marshmallow root if stools get too loose. Soaking chia seeds expand into a soothing gel coating intestines. Peppermint, ginger and fennel tea relieve bloating, as does massaging the gut. Enzyme supplements can ease the transition by helping break down fiber and FODMAPs from suddenly so much produce. Move your body gently every day, even just walking helps motility. And know this too shall pass!

The initial days feel challenging both physically and mentally as years of unhealthy food habits get dismantled and detoxed. But incredibly by Day 5, the light at the end of the tunnel appears – cravings fade, detox symptoms ease up, energy stabilizes. You start feeling lighter and cleaner, digestive issues resolve, mental clarity improves notably. Lean on group support, coping strategies and the Reset guidance to push through theshort yet intense healing crisis. The many proven benefits make the effort worthwhile – reduced inflammation, balanced hormones, reliable energy, normalized weight and mood, stronger gut health. Stay the course using approved ingredients as nourishment, knowing your future self with better living for decades ahead will thank you!

Tips To Fight Temptations and Stay Compliant

Here are 8 tactical tips to fight food temptations and stay compliant on the Clean Food Reset diet:

1. Prepare compliant grab-n-go snacks and meals so you always have Reset-friendly food accessible to avoid straying. Hard boil eggs, roast chicken breasts, cut up vegetables for quick snacks.

2. Drink water or herbal tea as the first response when any craving hits. We often misread thirst cues as hunger. Taking a short walk further helps with mindless mouth temptations.

3. Read labels vigilantly. Most packaged foods contain hidden sugar, seed oils and food additives which sabotage the program. Review banned ingredients list before each new purchase.

4. Buddy up with a friend, spouse or neighbor also doing the Reset. Having someone for social support, recipe exchange and cheating deterrent helps immensely.

5. Throw away trigger foods to avoid temptation staring from your pantry or fridge. Out of sight, out of mind. Donate the rest to food banks to avoid wastage. Block social media accounts showing non-compliant foods too for the month.

6. Start a daily gratitude practice for this new chance at optimal health. Being thankful for your body's healing stops deprivation mindset sneaking in.

7. If eating events crop up, offer to bring your own Reset compliant side so there is always a fallback safe dish. Prepare polite refusal phrases in advance for pushy friends.

8. When (not if) you slip up, forgive yourself immediately and resume program rules at the very next meal. Perfection is not the goal during this restart phase. Avoid spiraling into an all-day cheat bender after one mistake.

Every single meal is a chance to get back on track.

Stay vigilant amidst temptation especially through the first difficult week, deploying any of these bulletproof survival strategies. Your future vibrantly healthy self is worth all the temporary sacrifice. Those stubborn last 5 to 20 lbs will finally budge. Energy and mood lift clearly when food stops controlling your life. Most potently, you create sustainable habits for life free from the chains of chronic inflammation-driven illness small daily Surrenders set you back bit by bit until diagnosis day. Choose yourself; the Reset makes vibrant self-care possible!

Simple Clean Food Reset Recipes to Start Off

I won't pretend that cooking only from the approved ingredients list doesn't require more meal planning when you begin your Reset journey. But take heart that you can still create varied, delicious dishes beyond roasting plain chicken or whipping up another salad. In my years guiding clients through the 30-day elimination protocol, I've compiled easy yet satisfying recipes using Reset-friendly whole foods for their meals. I'll share my back pocket arsenal of go-to breakfasts, proteins, vegetable sides and even healthier desserts so your tastebuds never get bored.

Let's start the day strong with foundational recipes providing sustained energy minus inflammatory triggers setting off later cravings. Veggie-packed frittatas and crustless quiches are easy to adapt to your favorite produce combos and convenient for batch cooking. Simply wilt spinach, mushrooms and onions before adding whisked eggs and nut cheese to bake. Sweet potatoes lend natural sweetness for morning bowls or porridges paired with nuts, coconut and cinnamon. Overnight oats give future-you an effortless morning – combine chia seeds, almond milk and berries the night before. Or keep hard boiled eggs ready-to-peel as high protein snacks.

Incorporate gut-friendly resistant starches through white rice, potatoes or properly soaked beans. Let cooked then chilled white rice revive in flavorful fried rice with shrimp, peas, carrots and eggs. Roast red skin potatoes in coconut oil with onion and rosemary for potent phytonutrient sides or potato salad with fennel, apple cider vinegar and loads of parsley. Enjoy lectin-free lentil soup or white bean chicken chili simmered with vegetables for added prebiotics to feed good bacteria.

Speaking of which, fill half your plate at every meal with low-FODMAP veggies for nutritional powerhouses minus digestion issues. Beyond grazing yet another salad, get creative roasting cauliflower florets tossed in garlicky red pepper flakes and olive oil or cream up celery root mash akin to mashed potatoes. Fresh green beans sautéed with sliced almonds pair perfectly with fish entrees. I encourage clients to pick three colors of vegetables each meal to vary phytonutrients supporting detox processes.

Protein options branch beyond grilled chicken or fish fillets too. Wild caught salmon and tuna pack anti-inflammatory omega fats so I suggest recipes like pesto salmon with cashews or seared tuna over arugula. Pasture raised eggs shine so memorize how to whip up the perfect fluffy scramble or try frittatas baked in muffin tins for fast high protein snacks. Grass-fed meats like flank steak turn tender when marinated overnight in apple cider vinegar with rosemary and garlic. Ethical meats truly shine post Reset without needing heavy spice rubs or sugary sauces masking flavor.

Healthy fats provide sustained energy to stabilize blood sugar spikes without raising insulin so include options at each meal. Portion raw nuts or nut butter with apple slices, top salads with half an avocado or sneak extra virgin olive oil over roasted vegetables. Drizzle lemon tahini sauce on chicken skewers or salmon before baking. Blend full fat coconut milk into curry simmering with vegetables or add coconut butter for decadent hot drinks.

And yes you can even enjoy sweet treats that nourish minus blood sugar bombs! Chocolate avocado mousse, pumpkin custard baked with warming spices, or frozen banana blended into dairy-free nice cream prove you don't need inflammatory refined sugar to satisfy occasional dessert cravings. Berries blended into smoothies or chia pudding provide antioxidants too. Just pace portions without overindulging in natural sweeteners before your palate resets.

I invite you to get creative with approved whole foods tailored to your tastes so the 30 days don't feel restrictive. Set yourself up for success without deprivation sinking in by preparing Reset-friendly proteins, produce combos and even healthier desserts ready for easy assembling into satisfying meals. You'll discover an arsenal of recipes fueling your body's innate power to reverse illness while delighting your tastebuds along the way!

CHAPTER 3

A 30-Day Food Cleanse Rest Meal Plan

Here is a more detailed 30-day food cleanse diet plan including breakfast, lunch and dinner for each day:

Day 1:

Breakfast - Warm lemon water

Lunch - Fresh vegetable juice

Dinner - Vegetable broth

Day 2:

Breakfast - Fruit smoothie

Lunch - Mixed vegetable and fruit juice

Dinner - Green salad with vinaigrette

Day 3:

Breakfast - Melon

Lunch - Berries

Dinner - Baked apples

Day 4:

Breakfast - Steamed veggies

Lunch - Raw veggie salad

Dinner - Roasted vegetables

Day 5:

Breakfast - Ginger tea

Lunch - Vegetable broth

Dinner - Chamomile tea

Day 6:

Breakfast - Lentil sprout salad

Lunch - Mung bean sprout soup

Dinner - Chickpea sprouts hummus with celery sticks

Day 7:

Breakfast - Vegetable soup

Lunch - Mushroom soup

Dinner - Miso soup

Day 8:

Breakfast - Quinoa porridge with almond milk

Lunch - Millet salad

Dinner - Buckwheat stir fry

Day 9:

Breakfast - Soaked almonds

Lunch - Pumpkin seeds

Dinner - Sunflower seed pâté with flax crackers

Day 10:

Breakfast - Kale smoothie

Lunch - Berry smoothie

Dinner - Spinach smoothie

Day 11:

Breakfast - Lentil soup

Lunch - Chickpea salad

Dinner - Kidney bean chili

Day 12:

Breakfast - Brown rice porridge

Lunch - Quinoa salad

Dinner - Baked sweet potato and wild rice

Day 13:

Breakfast - Avocado toast

Lunch - Guacamole with raw veggies

Dinner - Zucchini pasta with olives

Day 14:

Breakfast - Green tea

Lunch - Chamomile tea

Dinner - Peppermint tea

Day 15:

Breakfast - Kefir

Lunch - Yogurt with blueberries

Dinner - Yogurt parfait

Day 16-29:

Follow same schedule repeating earlier days' meals

Day 30:

Slowly reintroduce unprocessed foods like eggs, fish, chicken, fruits, veggies, grains, nuts, seeds.

Understanding Your Body's Changes

The first week of any elimination diet feels challenging as years of physiological dependence gets dismantled. But stick through the short term intensity and your body soon stops reacting and responding to the constant influx of modern inflammatory foods. The change unmasks surprising benefits once symptoms attributed to "normal aging" disappear - effortless weight loss, balanced hormones, reliable mood and energy, better digestion and immunity.

Blood Sugar Regulation – Spiking glucose and insulin all day long from sugary, starchy foods stresses the pancreas eventually wearing it out. Just 72 hours into the Reset, participants are shocked by balanced energy sans crashes every few hours once digestive processes normalize. Even approved sweeteners must be minimized so taste buds reset and cravings fade. Stabilized blood sugar provides mental clarity too without urgent hunger hijacking concentration mid-morning or afternoon.

Hormone Balance – Dairy, soy and xenoestrogens in beauty & cleaning products hamper thyroid and reproductive hormones contributing to fatigue. They also disrupt cortisol stress responses and insulin sensitivity leading to stubborn weight gain. As these external influences get removed, the endocrine system finds homeostasis. Women breeze through menstruation finally instead of combatting PMS and period pain monthly with OTC medication bandaids.

Gut Health – Common irritants like gluten grains, lectins and inflammatory fats compromise intestinal lining integrity allowing undigested food particles and toxins leakage into the bloodstream. This provokes systemic inflammation eventually. Eliminating the worst offenders allows the gut to heal, tighten junctions and rebalance its microbiome population. Bloating, pain and bowel unpredictability reduce dramatically within days on the elimination diet as inflammation subsides.

Mental Health – Blood sugar swings and inflammation heighten anxiety, depression and motivation issues. Neurotransmitter precursors also get used up with nutrient-deficient modern foods in the diet. A week into the Reset, mood and focus transform for most people are neurotransmitters rebalance. Lightness from releasing years of stored toxins improves outlook as well. Many are able to reduce psychiatric medication dosages after eliminating mood saboteurs.

Detoxification – Toxic burdens accumulate from unhealthy dietary choices, environmental pollutants and stress hormones over years until organs like the liver and kidneys get overwhelmed. Removing inflammatory and high toxin-load foods while flooding your system with antioxidant and phytochemical-rich produce gives these organs an opportunity to reset, repair and restart natural detoxification pathways. Die-off reactions manifest temporarily as stored toxins exit.

Taste Changes – High salt, sugar and chemical flavors in processed convenience foods skew taste buds eventually requiring hyperpalatable combos to register as enjoyable. Just 2 weeks eliminating additives, health-harming oils and sweeteners recalibrates receptors. Vegetables, whole foods and simpler preparations become delicious again. Your microbiome shifts from craving high calorie processed items more towards fibrous fruits and vegetables.

The short term adjustment phase feels challenging yet treasured as self-inflicted issues get unmasked. Incredibly the actual food limitations matter far less than the exponential benefits – fast stubborn weight release, balanced hormones, reliable mood and energy, stronger digestion and sharper mental clarity. Elimination diets seem restrictive initially but actually free you from the real prison – living shackled to the whims of chronic illnesses and complaints you accepted as inevitable with age. The Reset reveals your body wants to be well as it sheds trapped toxins, inflammation and bloat once relieved of managing huge dietary burdens it was never designed for.

Recognizing Changes in Energy, Sleep, Mood, Etc.

The elimination diet intensely overhauls health as years of accumulated physiological burdens and toxins stored in tissues start releasing. Pay attention beyond just the number on your scale. Keep a journal tracking improvements in energy, mood, sleep, skin, digestion, mental clarity and more to stick with the program as your body cleanses and heals.

Energy – The first week feels exhausting between detox reactions and blood sugar crashes. But most participants cross a corner at days 8 to 10 where energy lifts higher and stabilizes between meals. This steady baseline sans urgent hunger, fatigue or cravings continues improving as mitochondria reawaken. Lightness pervades both physically and mentally without bloat, inflammation or toxins dragging you down. Exercise readiness and stamina may briefly reduce during the initial healing crisis before gradually surpassing previous capabilities.

Sleep – Tossing and turning from detox heat waves or night sweats impede deep sleep initially before regulation kicks in. But stick it out – the majority experience improved sleep quality with deeper REM cycles, more restorative rest needing less total hours, and consistent energy upon waking. Set yourself up for sleep success through the rollercoaster by avoiding exercise and food 3 hours before bedtime, limiting light and digital stimulation after dark, and sipping chamomile tea.

Mood – Difficult emotions and short fuses flare up by design during the first week as blood sugar drops between meals and your system detoxes. Support neurotransmitter balance with amino acid supplements like 5-HTP until cravings fade. But brace for awe as balanced energy transforms outlook. Lightness from releasing years of stored toxins and no longer managing debilitating symptoms every day lifts spirits and motivation exponentially. Future feels hopeful without illness dragging you down!

Digestion – Bloating and erratic bowel habits peak days 3 to 5 as years of waste clear out. Support gentle release with daily movement, digestive enzymes and herbs like marshmallow root for intestinal lining protection. Bloating and pain soon resolve as gut inflammation subsides sans irritants and microbiome diversity improves with wild ferments and fibrous fruits and veggies. Notice if heartburn, previously unrelenting, disappears after quitting trigger foods.

Skin, Hair & Nails – Acne surfaces initially as toxins exit through skin before complexion evens out. But persist because most experience dramatic skin improvements with better hydration, collagen formation and lowered inflammation levels. Scalp sheds old hair making way for stronger follicle regrowth. Nails thicken with improved protein and micronutrient absorption. Glowing from inside out becomes the new norm.

Mental Focus - Brain fog and distraction lift exponentially due to balanced blood sugar rather than urgent hunger hijacking concentration every few hours. Memory, quicker processing speed and motivation return. The instant energy and positivity infusion makes tasks requiring discipline or willpower far more achievable.

The rollercoaster first 10 days transitions quickly into steadier terrain by the halfway mark as your body adapts to consistent nourishment and sheds its former toxic burdens. Symptom cessation snowballs into genuine zest for life. Keep tracking positive changes in a journal for the moments you feel like quitting. Your future vibrant self is worth fighting for amidst the discomforts – lean on support, healthy distractions and trust the guidance until detox reactions shift into healing transformation!

Managing Ongoing Cravings and Learning True Hunger Signals

Cravings and hunger confusion sabotage even the most determined elimination diet efforts unless you deploy science-backed tricks to master internal cues. Tame temptations by understanding their emotional or physiological origins. Distinguish between physical hunger signalling actual caloric need versus mental urges for pleasure, stress relief or out of habit. Arm yourself with craving control tactics so you can respond appropriately to each trigger.

The hardest battle rages Days 3 to 5 when blood sugar normalizes before the body adapts to consistent nourishment all day. Lightheadedness, irritability, headaches and fatigue mimic urgent hunger signaling mealtime. Tame physiological triggers first by eating nutritious food every 4 to 5 hours, frontloading calories earlier in the day. Sip bone broth as a snack or drink herbal tea between meals to ride out waves. Add pink Himalayan salt for electrolytes, take magnesium and B vitamins to steady nerves.

Cravings also get loud when we actually crave emotional comfort, distraction from unpleasant tasks or relief from boredom and stress. Preempt emotional eating by scheduling activities, connecting with friends, trying meditation or Epsom salt baths for soothing. If you catch a craving, drink water first then do something engaging for 15 minutes before reevaluating if you require food. Often the intensity dies down once the underlying emotional need gets addressed or distraction shifts focus.

You absolutely require food for genuine stomach hunger signalling depleted reserves. Learn the distinct physiological signals like tummy rumbles, difficulty concentrating, irritability or headaches that manifest when blood sugar and nutrients run low. Keep Reset-approved proteins, fruits and vegetables accessible to fuel up promptly when those strike. Hard boiled eggs, carrots and nut butter make perfect hunger tamers.

Watch portion sizes with approved sweeteners and treats in early days before tastebuds normalize to simpler flavors. Eating too freely from these foods, even quality dark chocolate or fruit, activates reward centers driving further craving for sweets, salts and fats. Deal with oral fixation desires by brushing teeth after eating or chewing gum derived from xylitol birch bark.

Social eating and drinking events trip up even seasoned Food Resetter adherents. Politely decline temptation foods, bring approved dishes to share, focus on menu items you can partake in, or limit attendance time by having alternate plans shortly after. If you slip up, forgive yourself immediately without spiraling into punitive thinking or figure you've ruined the entire program. Every single meal presents a fresh opportunity to regain your footing with the very next Reset-aligned plate. Progress not perfection during this learning curve!

Arm yourself with knowledge of true hunger mechanisms – physical and emotional. Counter intense cravings most likely to ambush willpower between Days 3 to 5. Eat consistently every few hours from approved proteins, fruits and vegetables to ride out urges. Address underlying emotional needs without food to quiet a craving. You've totally got this! Stay the course and soon bingeing behavior lifts for good as you become resensitized to genuine hunger cues prompting when and how much to eat.

CHAPTER 4

Making the Clean Food Reset a Lifestyle

Congratulations, you made it! You should feel incredibly proud to have stuck with the intensive 30-day protocol. Now comes the exciting part as tangible improvements begin snowballing through renewed energy, balanced hormones, better digestion, easy weight management and heightened clarity. Key lessons start crystallizing that make adopting long term lifestyle modifications simple going forward.

First revel in the new normal – steady energy sans rollercoaster surges, crashes and cravings hijacking productivity. Stable blood sugar between satisfying meals roots you in each present moment without distraction. Inflammation plummets across organs, joints and digestive tract eliminating excuses around achy knees, acid reflux or brain fog sabotaging cognition. Even sleep consistency and mood stability start feeling effortless. This is your new vibrant baseline as chronic issues plaguing daily life for too long finally resolve with food triggers removed and nutrient reserves replenished.

Your tastebuds reset after a month sans flavor additives, sugars and refined oils. Vegetables, fruits and anti-inflammatory fats suddenly taste decadent. Time to savor natural flavors returns without shoveling meals down mindlessly between tasks. You adopt eating as self-care ritual tuning into your body's actual signals for hunger, fullness and satisfaction. Intuitive eating becomes possible once blood sugar levels out.

Equally potent, the identity shift takes hold as you stop self-identifying as the sick, inflamed, overweight victim of modernity. Through self-compassion yet dogged persistence removing dietary tripwires, you start acknowledging your inherent body wisdom designed for vitality First signs manifest as heightened confidence, motivation and optimism. Your future looks hopeful as illness no longer defines each day. Now you become a conscious, empowered agent co-creating your destiny through food choices honoring your vessel's needs.

So what next after the initial 30 days? The Reset makes adopting long term habit changes simple because you've witnessed such rapid benefits. Use the reintroduction phase to test previous inflammatory foods like gluten, dairy or coffee. You may tolerate ancient grains though modern hybridized wheat continues triggering issues. Goat dairy or ghee works for some folks. Just listen and learn your body's personal thresholds for potential irritants compared to eliminate foods.

This clarity makes it easier establishing sustainable healthy routines like consistent nutritious eating, stress-busting habits, restorative sleep and frequent movement versus sporadic crash diets. Ditch scales focusing solely on weight. Instead journal mood, energy, skin changes, period flow – tangible markers proving food directly impacts how you inhabit each day. When temptation arises, ask if a momentary food reward outweighs the gift of whole-body wellness now functioning optimally. Use that memory and self-compassion to realign choices.

You tackled the hardest part showing commitment simply through starting then sticking with the Reset when every neuron screamed for inflammatory yet familiar snacks. Now your momentum continues building because micronutrient resources fill your cells, toxic burdens lifted and organs strengthened to convert food properly into fuel. The tangible benefits make it easier to prioritize self-care tweaking recipes and lifestyle factors personalized for your unique biology. Congratulations committing to your highest potential vitality!

Forming Long-Term Habit Changes

Changing habits and forming new, healthier routines can be challenging. However, with commitment and consistency, it is possible to make lasting lifestyle changes. Here are some tips for forming long-term habit changes:

- Start small - Don't try to overhaul your entire life at once. Focus on one or two habits you want to change and take small, incremental steps. For example, if you want to eat healthier, start by eating one more serving of vegetables per day. Once that becomes routine, add another. Small changes are more sustainable over time.

- Make a plan - Decide what exactly you will do differently and make specific plans. State when, where, how and how often you will follow your new habit. Planning ahead helps turn good intentions into action. For example, commit to going to the gym 3 times per week on Monday, Wednesday and Friday at 7am before work.

- Prepare your environment - Remove temptations and make the new habit easy to accomplish. If you want to stop snacking unhealthily at night, remove junk food from your kitchen. If you want to exercise more, lay out your workout clothes and shoes the night before. A supportive environment facilitates success.

- Start a routine - Link the new habit to an existing routine to help remember it. For example, take your vitamins right after brushing your teeth in the morning. The established routine will serve as a reminder and cue for the new behavior.

- Track progress - Use a journal, calendar or app to record your habit changes. Tracking makes you more mindful of your behaviors and helps identify what's working. Checking off completed workouts or Xing out skipped sweets provides motivation.

- Enlist support- Tell friends and family about your new habit goal and ask them to cheer you on or even join you. Having a support system boosts commitment to change. Consider joining an online or in-person group related to your goal like a workout class or cooking club.

- Reward yourself - Celebrate achieving milestones related to your new habit. Treat yourself to a massage after a month of regular exercise or have your favorite dinner after a week without sweets. Positive reinforcement helps make the habit feel worthwhile.

- Be patient - It takes time for new habits to become automatic. Stick with your plan and allow at least a couple months for behaviors to fully take hold. Persistence through occasional slip ups leads to long-term change.

- Change your mindset - Adjust your thinking to view your new habit as an integral part of your identity rather than a chore. Reframe exercise as critical self-care instead of a task to check off. This mental shift helps cement new behaviors.

- Manage setbacks - Expect occasional backsliding and don't give up completely because of a few lapses. Analyze what led to the setback, develop a plan to get back on track, and implement it. One missed workout doesn't negate weeks of progress.

- Adjust as needed - Review your habit plan regularly and tweak where necessary. If your morning workout routine isn't sustainable, try switching to evenings. Refining your approach boosts your chances of making permanent change.

By starting small, planning thoroughly, and showing self-compassion through the ups and downs, you can turn positive intentions into lifelong habit change. Commitment and consistency are key, but don't forget to celebrate your wins along the way. The effort is well worth forming healthier habits that improve your quality of life.

Modifying the Program to Be Sustainable

When starting a new health program like diet, exercise or meditation, it's easy to go all in. You may be able to follow a strict routine for a while through sheer motivation. But for most people, rigid rules or intense habits are unsustainable long-term. The key is to implement changes in a flexible way that works for your lifestyle. Follow these tips to modify your program to make it more maintainable.

Start with small, incremental steps. Drastic changes in diet or two-hour daily workouts are hard to stick to. Make minor tweaks that seamlessly fit into your current routine. For example, if new to exercise, commit to a daily 20-minute walk instead of an intense cardio class. Or switch out soda for seltzer instead of eliminating all sweet drinks. Once the smaller change becomes habit, build on it.

Evaluate your schedule. Look at your current work and family commitments realistically. Aim for consistency even during busy times rather than intense efforts punctuated by lapses. For example, if work deadlines approach, maintain your gym routine but reduce sessions from one hour to 30 minutes. Or meal prep healthy batch recipes when time is short.

Focus on convenience. Make your program easy to follow, especially at first. Join a gym close to home or work. Have healthy snacks on hand. Streamline meal prep with simple recipes. Remove tempting junk food from your kitchen. Convenience facilitates consistency.

Build in flexibility. Allow yourself leeway, especially for special occasions. Attending a wedding or going on vacation makes strict dieting difficult. But exercise can be modified, like using the hotel gym. Expect setbacks and get back on track rather than abandoning your program.

Prioritize sustainability over speed. Gradual progress sustained over months and years beats rapid short-term results followed by burnout. Target steady weight loss of 1-2 pounds per week rather than crash dieting. Increase fitness level methodically and avoid injury.

Make it enjoyable. Habits are easier to maintain if you like doing them. Experiment to find physical activities you enjoy whether it's dance, martial arts or hiking. Discover new healthy recipes you genuinely crave. Mix up your workout routine to prevent boredom. Having fun keeps you motivated.

Listen to your body. Tune into your energy levels, aches and pains, sleep needs, stress levels and emotional state. Adjust your regimen accordingly to prevent exhaustion or burnout. You may need more rest days, better sleep hygiene or reduced intensity during high-stress periods.

Get support. Surround yourself with people who bolster your new healthy habits, not derail them. Consider joining classes and clubs related to your goals like a running group or cooking class. Having an exercise buddy or swapping recipes keeps you accountable.

Reevaluate regularly. Review your program every few weeks, especially when starting out. Make course corrections based on your progress, struggles and changing schedule. Adjusting along the way prevents relapse when life gets busy.

Developing sustainable habits takes some trial and error. But with a flexible mindset focused on the long-term, you can make lasting changes. Consistency over time trumps short-term intensity. Modify your approach to make your health program work realistically for your lifestyle.

CHAPTER 5

Clean Food Reset Recipes for Any Occasion

Building Routine Reset Meals

When doing a health reset, getting back to basics with simple, nourishing foods is key. Carefully planning reset breakfasts, lunches and dinners ensures you have healthy options on hand. Structure your meals around lean proteins, complex carbs, and plenty of fresh fruits and veggies. Here are some sample reset recipes to help build your daily routine:

Reset Breakfasts

Start your day right with a balanced reset breakfast. Good options provide protein for sustained energy along with fruits and whole grains.

Reset Omelet – Whip up a 3-egg white omelet with sautéed spinach and mushrooms, topped with avocado and salsa. Serve with a side of mixed berries.

Chia Seed Pudding – Combine chia seeds, almond milk, cinnamon, and chopped apples or berries. Soak overnight in the fridge to create a satisfying morning pudding.

Veggie Scramble – Sauté zucchini, peppers, onions, and greens. Scramble in 3 eggs or egg whites and add fresh tomato salsa. Pair with half an avocado and melon cubes.

Ancient Grain Porridge – Cook quinoa, amaranth, or buckwheat in almond milk with cinnamon, walnuts, and fresh peach slices for a warm cereal.

Green Smoothie – Blend banana, mango, spinach, chia seeds, almond butter, and almond milk for a nutrient packed drink.

Reset Lunches

Keep your midday meal light and energizing. Focus on lean proteins with veggie sides and fruit.

Turkey Lettuce Wraps – Wrap turkey, tomato, avocado and hummus in lettuce leaves for a simple assembled lunch. Enjoy with vegetable crudités and Greek yogurt dip.

Salmon Salad – Flake canned salmon over a bed of greens, chopped celery, shredded carrot, and cherry tomatoes. Drizzle with olive oil and balsamic vinaigrette.

Veggie Bowl – Fill a bowl with roasted sweet potato, beets, beans, avocado, and sautéed kale.

Tuna Salad – Mix tuna with chickpeas, celery, lemon juice, and Dijon. Serve alongside raw vegetables and apple slices.

Chicken Vegetable Soup – Simmer chicken breast, carrots, zucchini and spinach in broth. Pair with a small side salad.

Reset Dinners

In the evening, include lean protein and an array of vegetables for balanced nutrition.

Shrimp Buddha Bowl – Roast shrimp, cauliflower rice, broccoli, butternut squash, and chickpeas drizzled with tahini sauce for a complete meal in one bowl.

Sheet Pan Chicken – Roast chicken breast and vegetables like Brussels sprouts, carrots, and sweet potato all on one pan for easy cooking.

Vegetarian Chili – Make an easy hearty stew with beans, lentils, peppers, carrots, onions, and zucchini simmered in tomato sauce. Serve over quinoa or brown rice.

Taco Salad – Load salad greens with ground turkey or lean grass-fed beef, peppers, onions, avocado, salsa, and black beans for a Mexican inspired dinner.

Chicken & Vegetable Stir Fry – Quickly stir fry chicken strips, broccoli, mushrooms, bell peppers, carrots, and spinach. Serve over cauliflower rice.

Plan your reset meal routine ahead of time for the week. Prep basics like grains and proteins to keep on hand. With balanced nutrition locked in, you're set up for success all day long.

Easy Weeknight Meals and Hearty Weekend Dish Ideas

Streamlining Your Meals

Between work, family, and other obligations, it can be challenging to find time to prepare healthy meals. However, with some planning, it is possible to pull together nutritious dishes for weeknights and more indulgent fare on weekends. Follow these suggestions for effortless weekday meals and satisfying weekend recipe ideas.

Easy Weeknight Dinners

Keep your weeknight meals simple but nourishing. Focus on recipes with short prep times using versatile ingredients.

Sheet Pan Suppers – Toss protein and vegetables onto a baking sheet, season, and roast for a fuss-free dinner. Try combinations like salmon with green beans and potatoes or chicken thighs with squash and Brussels sprouts.

Eggs and Vegetables – Quickly sauté, scramble, or poach eggs and serve alongside sautéed greens, roasted veggies, or a spinach salad for an easy light dinner.

Baked Fish and Rice – Bake firm white fish like cod or tilapia topped with tomatoes, olives, and fresh herbs alongside baked or microwaved rice or grains.

Pasta and Salad – Boil pasta and mix with olive oil, garlic, veggies, greens, tuna, or white beans for fast nutrient-rich meals. Serve with a leafy side salad.

Soup and Sandwich – Pair canned or homemade vegetable/bean soup with a turkey, tuna, or veggie sandwich for cozy meals.

Hearty Weekend Recipes

On weekends when you have more time, prepare leisurely recipes that satisfy comfort food cravings. Invite friends and family over to share.

Brunch Casseroles – Assemble egg bakes, frittatas, and stratas the night before and bake the next morning for leisurely shared meals.

Roasts with Veggies – For unfussy feasts, roast beef, pork, or chicken in the oven along with potatoes, carrots, parsnips, and onions.

Chili or Stews – Slow cook hearty bean or meat-based chilis and stews that improve over hours or days in the fridge. Pair with crusty bread.

DIY Pizza Night – Set up a pizza bar with whole wheat dough, sauce, and toppings so everyone can customize their own healthy pies.

Taco/Fajita Bar – Grill meat and peppers/onions, provide tortillas, beans, rice, guacamole, salsa, and lettuce/cheese so guests can build Tex-Mex plates.

Pasta Bar – Boil a few shapes of pasta and set out sauces, vegetables, shrimp, chicken, meatballs, cheese, and garlic bread for DIY meals.

With go-to weeknight recipes and special weekend dishes in your repertoire, maintaining healthy homemade meals is totally doable. Get the whole family involved in preparing and customizing meals for added fun.

Holiday Meals, Parties, and Special Occasion Recipe

Holidays, parties, and special celebrations often center around tempting, indulgent foods. With some planning and creative recipes, you can still enjoy these occasions while maintaining your healthy eating habits. Follow these suggestions for nutrition-focused holiday meals, appetizers, and treats.

Holiday Meals

The main event meal often features traditional fare like turkey, ham, or roast beef with sides like mashed potatoes and gravy. Rethink classics with the following healthy swaps:

- Roast turkey or chicken with herbs instead of basting in butter or oil.

- Swap starchy potatoes or stuffing for roasted vegetables like Brussels sprouts, sweet potatoes, or butternut squash.

- Opt for fresh cranberry relish over heavy cranberry sauce.

- Make gravy with turkey stock instead of fat drippings.

- Choose whole grain rolls, wild rice, or quinoa instead of white potatoes or bread.

- Incorporate more vegetables like roasted green beans, asparagus, or sautéed spinach.

- For dessert, serve fresh fruit salad, poached pears, or baked apples rather than heavy pie or cake.

Party Appetizers

Avoid fatty chips, cheese platters, and fried finger foods. Bring healthier starters like:

- Fresh fruit and veggie platters with hummus or guacamole for dipping
- Smoked salmon on cucumber rounds
- Shrimp cocktail with lemon and hot sauce
- Turkey meatball skewers with chimichurri sauce
- Stuffed mushrooms or peppers
- Roasted chickpeas or nuts
- Edamame hummus in endive leaves

Special Occasion Treats

While it's fine to indulge, make room for desserts in your calorie budget and portion wisely. Bake lighter versions like:

- Poached pears or baked apples
- Meringue cookies or macaroons

- Fresh fruit tart on a whole grain crust

- Single layer cake or cupcakes

- Chocolate avocado mousse

- Single scoop sorbets or fruit sherbets

- Mixed berry compote over angel food cake

The key is moderating portions of traditional foods and adding healthier dishes. This allows you to still take part in the festivities while maintaining balance. Savor special occasion meals, but get right back on track with healthy habits afterwards.

Conclusion

In closing, adopting a clean food reset can truly transform your health and wellbeing for the better. What you put into your body on a daily basis provides the foundation for how you look, feel, and function. By filling your diet with natural, minimally processed foods like fruits, vegetables, lean proteins, whole grains, and healthy fats, you nourish your body with vital nutrients. Limiting added sugars, saturated fats, and excess sodium found in much of today's convenience food supports overall health.

Implementing a clean reset requires some lifestyle changes and initial effort. Meal planning, grocery shopping routines, and even kitchen setup may need adjustment to set yourself up for success. But with commitment to your goals and consistency with new habits, sustainable change is totally achievable. Supporting your body with clean, wholesome foods becomes second nature.

The clean food reset principles and meal plans provided throughout this book equip you with the knowledge and tools to transition to this beneficial way of eating. Whether your aim is weight loss, boosted energy, improved gut health or reduced inflammation, a clean diet can help you achieve results. By making thoughtful food choices and developing new kitchen skills, you take control over your health.

This lifestyle adjustment does far more than impact physical changes – it can enhance your whole outlook on life. The act of consciously caring for your body through nutritious food choices also has mental and emotional benefits. You feel more empowered, motivated, and in tune with your body's needs. Making positive strides with your health builds confidence and self-esteem.

Commit to your wellbeing starting today. Take that first step towards clean eating and experience the incredible impacts it can have on your life. You have the ability to become the healthiest version of yourself through the power of food.